SLOW

DIET

Slow Cooker: The Easy and Healthy Ketogenic Recipes
for Your Slow Cooker

Healthy Cooking for Weight Loss

@ Jesse Wells

Published By Adam Gilbin

@ Jesse Wells

Slow Cooker: The Easy and Healthy Ketogenic Recipes
for Your Slow Cooker

Healthy Cooking for Weight Loss

All Right RESERVED

ISBN 978-1-990053-55-9

TABLE OF CONTENTS

One Pot Chicken And Gravy 1

Orange Chicken 3

Orange Cinnamon Chicken 5

Orange Cranberry Chicken 7

Orange Glazed Chicken Breasts... 9

Orange Teriyari Chicken 11

Pizza Chicken 13

Provencale Chicken Supper 15

Quick N Easy Mushroom Chicken 17

Roast Chicken 18

Saucy Chicken Thighs 19

Southwestern Chicken Stew.. 20

Soy Chicken 21

Swiss Chicken Casserole 23

Barbecue Chicken.. 25

Cheese Crockpot Chicken... 26

Easy Pork Chops 27

Cinnamon Pork Stew 29

Pork & Sausage Stew.. 31

Pork Roast With Green Chilies 33

Mediterranean Beef With Artichokes 35

Mediterranean Braised Beef... 37

Beef Stew With Mariana Sauce....................................... 39

Beef & Vegetable Stew.. 40

Mediterranean Pot Roast... 42

Sweet Brussels Sprouts 44

Nuts Black Beans Mix 45

Onion Broccoli Mix.. 46

Tender Bean Medley.. 47

Honey Green Beans Mix.. 49

Green Onions With Creamy Chicken............................... 50

Marjoram Peas And Carrots 51

Garlic Cauliflower Pilaf 53

Squash Salad... 54

Spinach Salad 56

Chicken In Sun Dried Tomato Sauce 57

Crock Pot Whole Chicken 58

Corn, Mushrooms Chicken Stew 59

Pork White Bean Chili 60

Chicken And Baby Carrots Stew 61

Pork Meat Stew 62

Moroccan Lamb, Tomato Sauce & Green Peppers Stew 63

Mexican Lamb Chili 64

Pork, Mushrooms & Herbs Stew 66

Two Beans Chili 67

Chicken Green Curry 69

Chicken & Artichoke Hearts 71

Green Peppers, Chicken And Green Onions 72

Haitian Spinach Shrimp Stew 73

Black Bean Chicken Chili 74

Duck Curry 76

Tandoori Paneer Tikka Masala 77

Tandoori Masala Spice Mix 82

Tandoori Masala Spice Mix 84

Masala Beef With Ginger And Curry Leaf........................ 86

Jonagold's Chicken Vindaloo 90

Grilled Chicken Thighs Tandoori...................................... 94

Indian Tandoori Chicken.. 97

Tandoori Paneer Tikka Masala 100

Root Vegetable, Barley, Kale & Sausage Stew (Paleo) . 105

Crockpot Jambalaya Soup (Paleo) 107

Perfectly Cooked Yams (Paleo) 110

Pulled Pork Waffle Burgers (Paleo) 111

Crockpot Sweet Potato Basil Soup (Paleo).................... 115

Sausage And Peppers 117

Sausage Breakfast Casserole 119

Sausage Ratatouille 121

Rosemary And Thyme Roast Lamb................................ 123

Moroccan Lamb Stew... 125

Indian Curried Lamb... 127

Spiced Stuffed Apples... 129

Pumpkin Pudding 131

Berry Crumble 133

Tomatoes And Kidney Beans........................... 135

Chicken Tacos.. 137

Chicken Creole... 139

Mu Shu Turkey 141

Chicken Casserole.. 143

Minestrone Stew 144

Green Chili Stuffed Chicken Breasts.............. 146

Honeyed Chicken Wings................................. 148

Lemon Tarragon Chicken................................ 149

Low-Fat Chicken & Veggie Bake 150

Maple Barbecue Chicken................................ 151

Mediterranean Chicken.................................. 152

One Pot Chicken Gravy................................... 154

Orange Burgundy Chicken.............................. 156

Provincial Chicken 157

Russian Chicken... 159

Spaghetti Sauce With Chicken & Sausage 160

Spanish Chicken 162

Spicy Chicken Wings 163

Sweet 'N' Sour Chicken 164

Teriyaki Sauce Wings 166

Masala Beef & Rice 168

Mediterranean Beef & Pasta 170

Beef, Zucchini, & Eggplant Stew 172

Herbed Beef Stew 174

Tuscan Beef Stew 176

Mediterranean Eggplant 178

Greek Style Eggplant 180

Lebanese Eggplant Stew 182

Eggplant & Tomato Sauce 184

Italian Style Mushrooms 186

One Pot Chicken And Gravy

Ingredients:

- 1 packaged baby carrots

- 1 can cream of chicken soup

- 1 packaged dry onion soup mix

- Boneless, skinless chicken breasts

- Potatoes, quartered, with jackets

- About 6 stalks celery

Directions:

1. Line the bottom the Crockpot with Veggies.
2. Brown chicken breasts in PAM or vegetable spray.
3. Lay the browned chicken over vegetables.
4. Pour the cream of chicken soup, over the chicken.
5. Sprinkle with dry onion soup mix.

6. Cover and cook for 12 hours on low, or 6 hours on high.

Orange Chicken

Ingredients:

- 8 ounces Frozen concentrate orange juice

- 2 cups Shredded coconut

- 2 cups Orange segments or canned, mandarin oranges

- 2 Green onions, chopped

- 6 Chicken breasts boned and skinned

- 1 teaspoon Ginger

- 1 teaspoon Salt

- Pepper

Directions:

1. Place chicken, ginger, salt, pepper and frozen orange juice in crock pot and cook on low 6 hours.

2. Once ready, top with coconut, orange segments and green onions.
3. Serve chicken on hot cooked rice.

Orange Cinnamon Chicken

Ingredients:

- 1/2 Pound Butter

- 2 Cups Orange juice

- 1/2 Teaspoon Cinnamon

- Salt and pepper to taste

- 4 Pounds Chicken pieces

- 1 Cup Chicken broth

- 1 Cup Raisins or sultanas

- 1 Tablespoon Flour

Directions:

1. Heat butter in a skillet, and brown chicken on all sides.
2. Once brown, place the chicken in the Slow cooker.

3. Mix all other Ingredients:, except flour, in skillet.
4. Stir well and pour over chicken.
5. Cover and cook on LOW for 4 to 6 hours.
6. Remove one cup of sauce from pot and mix with flour, mixing well.
7. Pour the sauce flour mixture back into the pot.
8. Turn pot on HIGH and cook and additional half hour.
9. Serve

Orange Cranberry Chicken

Ingredients:

- 8 chicken breast halves , boned, skinned

- 1/2 cup orange juice

- 2 tablespoons melted butter or margarine

- 1 orange, sliced

- 1 cup chopped fresh cranberries

- 2 tablespoons brown sugar

- 5 slices cinnamon-raisin bread

- 2 tablespoons melted margarine or butter

- 1/2 teaspoon grated orange peel

Directions:

1. In medium bowl, mix cranberries and brown sugar; set aside.
2. Toast bread, chop into 1/2-inch cubes.

3. Mix bread cubes, 2 TBL melted butter, orange peel and cranberry mixture.

4. After placing in a small plastic bag, pound all chicken breasts with a meat mallet, one at a time.

5. Pour about 1 cup cranberry mixture on center of each chicken breast and roll up.

6. In shallow dish, mix orange juice and 2 tablespoons melted butter.

7. Roll filled chicken breasts in orange-juice mixture until completely coated.

8. Place the tolled and coated chicken breasts in slow cooker.

9. Cover and cook on LOW about 5 hours.

10. Garnish with orange slices and serve.

Orange Glazed Chicken Breasts

Ingredients:

- 2 Tbls. cornstarch

- 6 (6-oz) chicken breast halves

- 1/5 Cup water

- 1 (6-oz) frozen orange juice concentrate

- 1 tsp. dried marjoram leaves

Directions:

1. Mix thawed orange juice and marjoram in shallow dish.
2. Immerse each breast in orange juice mixture and place in the crock pot.
3. Pour remaining sauce over breasts.
4. Cover and cook on low 7-9 hours or on high for 4-5 hours.
5. Before serving, take out the chicken breasts from crock pot.

6. Combine water and cornstarch in the sauce mixture and cook covered on high for about 15-30 minutes.

7. Pour the thickened mixture over chicken and serve.

Orange Teriyari Chicken

Ingredients:

- One 16 ounce package loose-pack frozen broccoli, baby carrots, and water chestnuts

- 2 tbsp. quick-cooking tapioca

- 1 pound skinless, boneless chicken breast halves or thighs

Sauce:

- 1 tsp. finely shredded orange peel

- 1 tsp. ground ginger

- Cut chicken into 1" pieces.

- 1 cup chicken broth

- 2 tbsp. brown sugar

- 2 tbsp. teriyaki sauce

- 1 tsp. dry mustard

Directions:

1. Lay the vegetables at the bottom of the Crockpot.
2. Sprinkle tapioca over veggies.
3. Put chicken on top of that.
4. Mix sauce Ingredients: and pour over chicken.
5. Cover and cook on low for 4-6 hours or on high for 2-3. Serve with rice.

Pizza Chicken

Ingredients:

- 2 tablespoons tomato paste

- 1 cup water

- 1 tablespoon dried parsley

- 1 tablespoon dried oregano

- 1 tablespoon dried basil

- 1 bay leaf

- salt and pepper to taste

- 4 skinless, boneless chicken breasts, cut into bite size pieces

- 1 onion, chopped

- 1 green bell pepper, chopped

- 2 stalks celery, sliced

- 1 (10.75 ounce) can condensed tomato soup

- 1 (10.75 ounce) can condensed cream of mushroom soup

Directions:

1. Put the chicken, onion, bell pepper and celery in a slow cooker.
2. Mix the tomato soup, cream of mushroom soup, tomato paste, water, parsley, oregano, basil, salt and pepper in a bowl.
3. Stir thoroughly and pour mixture over chicken and vegetables in slow cooker.
4. Stir to completely cover the chicken and add bay leaf.
5. Cook on Low setting for 8 hours.

Provencale Chicken Supper

Ingredients:

- 1 cup diced yellow bell pepper

- 1 (16oz) can navy beans, rinsed and drained

- 1 (14oz) can pasta-style chunky tomatoes, undrained

- 4 (6oz) chicken breasts, skinless & boneless

- 2 tsp dried basil

- 1/2 tsp salt, divided

- 1/2 tsp pepper, divided

Directions:

1. Lay the chicken in slow cooker and season with basil, 1 tsp salt and 1 tsp pepper.
2. Mix the left over salt, pepper, bell pepper, beans and tomatoes in bowl and stir well.
3. Pour the mixture over chicken.

4. Cover and cook on high for 1 hour and then on low for 5 hours.
5. Pour bean mixture into 4 shallow bowls.
6. In each of the 4 bowls, put 1 breast and 3/4 cup bean mixture. Serve.

Quick N Easy Mushroom Chicken

Ingredients:

- 1 chicken bouillon cube, crushed

- 1 can cream of mushroom soup

- 1 c. boiling water

- 4 Chicken Breasts

- 4 medium potatoes, peeled and chunked

- 4-5 carrots, peeled and sliced

Directions:

1. Put the chicken in crock pot and encircle with potatoes and carrots.
2. Combine remaining Ingredients: in a separate bowl.
3. Pour into the Crockpot, covering everything.
4. Cook on low 6-8 hours
5. Serve with rolls on the side.

Roast Chicken

Ingredients:

- dried seasoning, i.e. oregano, basil, rosemary, etc.

- butter

- 1 whole chicken

- salt & pepper

- parsley

Directions:

1. Wash chicken well.
2. Season cavity with salt, pepper and parsley.
3. Place in crock pot breast side up.
4. Season the top with a little salt, pepper, and seasoning of your choice.
5. Layer breast with butter.
6. Cook on high one hour and low for 10-12 hours. Serve.

Saucy Chicken Thighs

Ingredients:

- 2 cloves minced garlic

- salt and pepper to taste

- 1 tsp Italian Seasoning

- 3 lbs bone in/skinless chicken thighs

- 1 can Italian style diced tomatoes

- I can tomato sauce

- 1 chopped onion

Directions:

1. Place all Ingredients: in crock pot and cook on high 1 hour then low 6 hours.
2. Serve with rice.

Southwestern Chicken Stew

Ingredients:

- 2 cans cream of mushroom or cream of chicken soup

- 2 cans of corn or one bag of frozen corn

- About 2 cups of water or chicken broth

- About 3 boneless skinless chicken breasts

- 1 can Rotel tomatoes

- 1 can black beans or 1 can of red beans

Directions:

1. Place all Ingredients: in Crockpot. (Pour the contents of all cans without draining)
2. Cook on low for about 8 hours. Serve.

Soy Chicken

Ingredients:

- 2-4 carrots

- 1 an onion, chopped

- 6 whole garlic cloves

- 1 tsp oregano

- seasonings of your choosing

- 1 tbls oil

- 1 whole chicken, cut into 8 pieces

- 2 c chicken broth

- 1/2 c soy sauce

- 1/2 c Worcestershire sauce

- 5 or 6 small to med sized potatoes (or as many as you want/need that will fit)

Directions:

1. In a skillet, heat oil and brown chicken on all sides.
2. Cut potatoes into bite size pieces, dice carrots and onion.
3. Lay the veggies, including garlic cloves, at the bottom of the Crockpot.
4. Add in seasonings, soy and Worcestershire sauce and stir well.
5. Place the Chicken on top.
6. Cook on high for about 5 hrs, or on low for about 8-10 hours.Serve.

Swiss Chicken Casserole

Ingredients:

- 1 can cream of mushroom soup

- 1/2 cup milk

- 2 cups stuffing mix

- 1 cup butter or margarine, melted

- 6 chicken breasts, boneless and skinless

- 6 slices Swiss cheese

Directions:

1. Coat the Crockpot with Cooking Spray.
2. Put the chicken breasts in pot.
3. Put cheese on top of the Chicken Breasts.
4. Mix soup and milk, stirring thoroughly and pour into Crockpot.
5. Pour cheese and stuffing mix over the chicken.
6. Sprinkle melted butter over stuffing mix.

7. Cook on low 8 to 10 hours or high 4 to 6 hours.

Barbecue Chicken

Ingredients:

- 3/4 cup brown sugar

- 3 tablespoons Worcestershire sauce

- 1 Chicken, cut up and skin removed

- 1 cup ketchup

Directions:

1. Lay the chicken in Crockpot.
2. Mix remaining Ingredients: and pour over chicken.
3. Cook 4 hours on high or 8-10 hours on low.

Cheese Crockpot Chicken

Ingredients:

- 2 cans cream chicken soup

- 1 can chedder cheese soup

- 3 whole boneless and skinless chicken breasts

Directions:

1. Season the Chicken Creasts with salt, pepper and garlic powder.
2. Place in crockpot and pour the three soups directly from the cans.
3. Cover and cook for 8-10 hours.
4. Serve over rice or noodles.

Easy Pork Chops

Ingredients:

- 1 teaspoon poultry seasoning

- 1 tablespoon garlic powder

- 2 garlic cloves, minced

- 1 teaspoon paprika

- 4 pork chops, thick cut, boneless

- 1/2 cup olive oil

- 1 cup chicken broth

- 1 teaspoon basil, dried

- 1 teaspoon oregano, dried

Directions:

1. Season pork chops with salt and pepper and place into the slow cooker

2. Add all remaining Ingredients:

3. Cover and cook for 8 hours on LOW

Cinnamon Pork Stew

Ingredients:

- 1 teaspoon thyme, dried

- 1 teaspoon cinnamon, ground

- 1 tablespoon honey

- 4 ounces feta cheese, crumbled

- 2 pounds pork loin, boneless, cut into cubes

- 2 cups pearl onions

- 14.5 ounces can chicken broth

- 2 cup dry red wine

- 1/3 cup flour

Directions:

1. In the slow cooker, add pork, thyme, flour, and cinnamon. Toss well and add balsamic vinegar, red wine, onion, honey, and broth

2. Cover and cook for 9 hours on LOW

3. Add cheese and serve

Pork & Sausage Stew

Ingredients:

- 6 carrots, sliced

- 2 garlic cloves, minced

- 2 cups onion, chopped

- 3 tablespoons tomato paste

- 1 teaspoon black pepper, ground

- 2 teaspoons thyme, fresh, crushed

- 2 pounds pork shoulder, cut into bite size cubes

- 16 ounces polish sausage, sliced

- 1 cup cherry tomatoes, halved

- 14 ounces can chicken broth, reduced sodium

- 2 (15 ounces each) cannellini beans, rinsed, drained

31

Directions:

1. In the slow cooker, add all Ingredients: except cherry tomatoes

2. Cover and cook for 10 hours on LOW

3. Add cherry tomatoes and cook for 10 minutes

Pork Roast With Green Chilies

Ingredients:

- 1 cup chicken broth

- 1 cup cilantro, chopped

- 1 tablespoon lime juice, fresh

- 1/8 teaspoon each; kosher salt and ground black pepper

- ½ teaspoon cumin, ground

- 2 pounds pork roast

- 10 ounces can tomatoes with green chilies

- 15 ounces can diced green chilies

- 1 yellow onion, peeled, diced

- 1 sweet potato, peeled, diced

Directions:

1. In the slow cooker, add all Ingredients: except cilantro and lime juice

2. Cook for 7 hours on LOW

3. Drizzle with lime juice and garnish with cilantro

Mediterranean Beef With Artichokes

Ingredients:

- 1 teaspoon cumin, ground
- 1 teaspoon basil, dried
- 1 teaspoon parsley, dried
- 1 teaspoon oregano, dried
- 4 garlic cloves, minced
- 1 onion, diced
- 1 tablespoon grapeseed oil
- 14 ounces can artichoke hearts, drained, halved
- 32 fluid ounces container beef broth
- 2 pounds stewing beef
- 1 cup Kalamata olives, pitted, chopped
- 15 ounces can diced tomatoes
- 1 bay leaf

Directions:

1. Add oil in a skillet and heat over medium-high
2. Cook beef until browned. Transfer to the slow cooker
3. Add all remaining Ingredients:
4. Cover and cook for 7 hours on LOW

Mediterranean Braised Beef

Ingredients:

- 1 teaspoon pepper

- 4 shallots, sliced

- 2 onions, sliced

- 1 teaspoon salt

- 1 teaspoon pepper

- 3 pounds chuck roast

- 1/2 cup balsamic vinegar

- 1/2 cup dates, pitted, chopped

- 1/2 cup all purpose flour

- 1 cup water

- 1 teaspoon salt

Directions:

1. Coat beef with flour and place into the slow cooker

2. Add all remaining Ingredients:

3. Cover and cook for 8 hours on LOW

Beef Stew With Mariana Sauce

Ingredients:

- 1 teaspoon basil, dried

- 1 teaspoon oregano, dried

- 2 cups marinara sauce

- 2 pounds beef stew, cut into cubes

- 16 ounces jar drained artichoke hearts

- 1 onion, diced

Directions:

1. In the slow cooker, add all Ingredients:
2. Cover and cook for 7 hours on LOW setting

Beef & Vegetable Stew

Ingredients:

- 4 thyme sprigs, fresh
- 2 cup all purpose flour
- 2 pounds beef chuck roast, trimmed, cut into bite size cubes
- 2 tablespoons garlic powder
- 16 ounces can cremini mushrooms, sliced
- 28 ounces can whole tomatoes, peeled
- 4 large carrots, chopped
- 2 cups vegetable broth
- 2 sprigs rosemary, fresh

Directions:

1. In a bowl, add garlic powder and flour. Mix well

2. Season meat with salt and pepper, coat with flour and garlic powder mixture, and cook in hot oil until browned.

3. Transfer to the slow cooker

4. Add red onion, garlic, carrot, red wine, tomato, rosemary, thyme, and vegetable broth

5. Cover and cook for 5 hours on HIGH

6. Add mushrooms, cover, and cook for an additional 30 minutes

Mediterranean Pot Roast

Ingredients:

- 1 garlic clove, chopped

- 1 tablespoon Italian seasoning

- 1 teaspoon salt

- 3 pounds beef chuck roast, boneless

- 1 pound bag pearl onions

- 1/3 cup sun dried tomatoes, chopped

- 1 cup beef broth

- 1 cup Kalamata olives, pitted, sliced

Directions:

1. Heat a nonstick skillet over medium-high
2. Season beef with Italian seasoning and salt, cook until browned in the skillet.
3. Transfer to the slow cooker

4. Add onions, olives, tomatoes, and broth

5. Cover and cook for 6 hours on LOW

Sweet Brussels Sprouts

Ingredients:

- 1 tablespoon olive oil

- 2 tablespoons maple syrup

- 1 tablespoon thyme, chopped

- 1 pounds Brussels sprouts, trimmed and halved

- 2 tablespoons mustard

- 1 cup vegetable stock

Directions:

1. In your slow cooker, mix the sprouts with the mustard and the other Ingredients:, toss, put the lid on and cook on Low for 3 hours.

2. Divide between plates and serve as a side dish.

Nuts Black Beans Mix

Ingredients:

- 1 tablespoon lime juice

- 2 tablespoons cilantro, chopped

- 2 tablespoons pine nuts

- 1 pound black beans, soaked overnight and drained

- 1 cup vegetable stock

Directions:

1. In your slow cooker, mix the beans with the stock and the other Ingredients:, toss, put the lid on and cook on Low for 6 hours.
2. Divide everything between plates and serve.

Onion Broccoli Mix

Ingredients:

- 1 teaspoon Worcestershire sauce

- 1/2 cup yellow onion, chopped

- 2 tablespoons olive oil

- 6 cups broccoli florets

- 1 and 2 cups cheddar cheese, shredded

- 1 cup coconut cream

Directions:

1. In a bowl, mix broccoli with coconut cream, cheese, onion, and Worcestershire sauce, toss and transfer to your Slow cooker.
2. Add olive oil, toss again, cover, and cook on High for 2 hours.
3. Serve as a side dish.

Tender Bean Medley

Ingredients:

- 2 bay leaves

- 16 ounces kidney beans, drained

- 15 ounces canned black-eyed peas, drained

- 15 ounces canned northern beans, drained

- 15 ounces canned corn, drained

- 15 ounces canned lima beans, drained

- 15 ounces canned black beans, drained

- 2 celery ribs, chopped

- 1 green bell pepper, chopped

- 1 yellow onion, chopped

- 1 sweet red pepper, chopped

- 1 cup honey

- 1 cup Italian dressing

- 1 cup of water

- 1 tablespoon cider vinegar

Directions:

1. In your Slow cooker, mix celery with red and green bell pepper, onion, honey, Italian dressing, water, vinegar, bay leaves, kidney beans, black-eyed peas, northern beans, corn, lima beans, and black beans, stir, cover, and cook on Low for 5 hours.

2. Divide between plates and serve as a side dish.

Honey Green Beans Mix

Ingredients:

- 1 cup olive oil

- 2 teaspoon soy sauce, low sodium

- 16 ounces green beans

- 1 cup honey

Directions:

1. In your Slow cooker, mix green beans with honey, olive oil, soy sauce, stir, cover, and cook on Low for 2 hours.
2. Divide between plates and serve as a side dish.

Green Onions With Creamy Chicken

Ingredients:

- 1/2 cup honey

- 2 cups chicken fillet, minced

- 2 tablespoons green onions, chopped

- 1 cup organic almond milk

- 3 tablespoons olive oil

- 2 cups coconut cream

Directions:

1. In your Slow cooker, mix all Ingredients: and cook on Low for 4 hours.
2. Stir the cooked meal, divide between plates and serve as a side dish.

Marjoram Peas And Carrots

Ingredients:

- 1/2 cup of water

- 1/2 cup honey

- 4 garlic cloves, minced

- 1 teaspoon marjoram, dried

- 1 yellow onion, chopped

- 1 pound carrots, sliced

- 16 ounces peas

- 1/2cup olive oil

Directions:

1. In your Slow cooker, mix the onion with carrots, peas, olive oil, water, honey, garlic, and marjoram, cover, and cook on Low for 5 hours.

2. Stir peas and carrots mix, divide between plates and serve as a side dish.

Garlic Cauliflower Pilaf

Ingredients:

- 2 garlic cloves, minced

- 1 pound Portobello mushrooms, sliced

- 2 cups warm water

- 1 cup cauliflower rice

- 6 green onions, chopped

- 3 tablespoons ghee, melted

Directions:

1. In your Slow cooker, mix cauliflower rice with green onions, melted ghee, garlic, mushrooms, water, stir well, cover, and cook on Low for 3 hours.
2. Divide between plates and serve as a side dish.

Squash Salad

Ingredients:

- 1 garlic clove, minced

- 1 big butternut squash, peeled and cubed

- 1/2 teaspoon ginger, grated

- 1 teaspoon cinnamon powder

- 3 cups of coconut milk

- 1 tablespoon olive oil

- 1 cup carrots, chopped

- 1 yellow onion, chopped

- 1 teaspoon honey

- 1 and 2 teaspoons curry powder

Directions:

1. In your Slow cooker, mix oil with carrots, onion, honey, curry powder, garlic, squash,

ginger, cinnamon, and coconut milk, stir well, cover, and cook on Low for 4 hours.

2. Stir, divide between plates, and serve as a side dish.

Spinach Salad

Ingredients:

- 3 garlic cloves, minced

- 10 ounces vegetable stock

- 6 ounces baby spinach

- 3 pounds butternut squash, peeled and cubed

- 1 yellow onion, chopped

- 2 teaspoons thyme, chopped

Directions:

1. In your Slow cooker, mix squash cubes with onion, thyme, and stock, stir, cover, and cook on Low for 4 hours.

2. Transfer squash mixture to a bowl, add spinach, toss, divide between plates and serve as a side dish.

Chicken In Sun Dried Tomato Sauce

Ingredients:

- a pinch of dried thyme and oregano

- 2 tbsp. coconut oil

- Salt and ground black pepper to taste

- 4 pounds dark chicken meat

- 12 sun dried tomatoes, chopped

- 1 cup coconut cream or full fat coconut milk

- 1 cup chicken broth

- 1/2 cup white wine (optional)

Directions::

1. Put Ingredients: in the slow cooker.
2. Cover, and cook on low for 7 to 9 hours.

Crock Pot Whole Chicken

Ingredients:

- 1 cup chopped parsnip (optional)

- 2 cups chopped onions

- 2 tbsp. coconut oil

- 1 whole chicken with skin on

- 1 cup sliced celery

- 1 cup chopped carrot

- Rub paprika, salt and ground black pepper on the chicken skin and inside. Optionally add lemon quarters inside.

Directions::

1. Put veggies in the slow cooker and place chicken on top.

2. Cover, and cook on low for 7 to 9 hours.

Corn, Mushrooms Chicken Stew

Ingredients:

- 2 cups sliced mushrooms

- 1 cups chopped onions

- 1 cup corn (optional)

- 2 tbsp. coconut oil

- 2 cups tomato paste

- Salt and ground black pepper to taste

- 4 pounds chicken meat

Directions::

1. Put Ingredients: in the slow cooker.
2. Cover, and cook on low for 7 to 9 hours.

Pork White Bean Chili

Ingredients:

- 1 cup sweet corn (optional)

- Salt, ground black pepper and ground cumin to taste

- 2-3 cups beef stock

- 4 pounds minced pork meat

- 2 cups sliced red peppers

- 1 cup chopped onions

- 2 tbsp. coconut oil

- 1 cup uncooked cannellini beans

- 1/4 cup sliced jalapeno peppers (adjust heat to taste)

Directions::

1. Put Ingredients: in the slow cooker.
2. Cover, and cook on low for 7 to 9 hours.

Chicken And Baby Carrots Stew

Ingredients:

- 2 tbsp. coconut oil

- Salt, ground black pepper to taste

- 4 pounds dark chicken meat

- 1 & 1/2 cups baby carrots

- 1 cup chopped onions

Directions::

1. Put Ingredients: in the slow cooker.
2. Cover, and cook on low for 7 to 9 hours.

Pork Meat Stew

Ingredients:

- 1 bunch chopped parsley

- Salt, ground black pepper and ground cumin to taste

- 1 cup beef stock

- 4 pounds cubed pork meat

- 2 tomatoes, sliced

- 1 cup chopped onions

- 2 tbsp. coconut oil

- 2 large red peppers, sliced

Directions::

1. Put Ingredients: in the slow cooker.
2. Cover, and cook on low for 7 to 9 hours.

Moroccan Lamb, Tomato Sauce & Green Peppers Stew

Ingredients:

- 2 cups tomato paste

- 3 cups green peppers

- 2 Tbsp. minced garlic.

- 2 Tbsp. ground cumin.

- 2 cups chopped onions

- 2 tbsp. coconut oil

- Salt, ground black pepper to taste

- 4 pounds lamb meat, cubed

Directions::

1. Put Ingredients: in the slow cooker.
2. Cover, and cook on low for 8 hours.

Mexican Lamb Chili

Ingredients:

- 2 tbsp. cumin seeds

- 1 tsp. ground cayenne pepper

- 1 tsp. ground coriander

- 1 tsp. salt

- 3 cups cooked kidney beans

- 2-3 fresh hot chili peppers, chopped

- 2 tbsp. coconut oil

- 2 onions, chopped

- 3 cloves garlic, minced

- 3 pounds cubed lamb meat

- 1 cup corn

- 1 cup tomato paste

- 2 cups beef broth

Directions::

1. Put Ingredients: in the slow cooker.

2. Cover, and cook on low for 8 hours.

Pork, Mushrooms & Herbs Stew

Ingredients:

- 4 pounds pork shoulder

- 3 cups sliced mushrooms

- 1/2 cup each parsley, cilantro and dill

- 2 Tbsp. minced garlic.

- 2 cups chopped onions

- 2 tbsp. coconut oil

- Salt, ground black pepper to taste

Directions::

1. Put Ingredients: in the slow cooker.
2. Cover, and cook on low for 8 hours.

Two Beans Chili

Ingredients:

- 2 cups beef broth

- 1 tbsp. cumin seeds

- 1 tsp. dried oregano

- 1 tsp. ground cayenne pepper

- 1 tsp. ground coriander

- 1 tsp. salt

- 3 cups cooked kidney beans

- 3 cups cooked navy beans

- 4 fresh hot chili peppers, chopped

- 2 tbsp. coconut oil

- 2 onions, chopped

- 3 cloves garlic, minced

- 1 pound ground beef

- 3/4 pound beef sirloin, cubed

- 2 cups diced tomatoes

- 1 cup strong brewed coffee

- 1 cup tomato paste

Directions::

1. Put Ingredients: in the slow cooker.

2. Cover, and cook on low for 4 hours.

Chicken Green Curry

Ingredients:

- 4 pounds chicken meat

- 2 cups sliced veggies (green beans and green peppers)

- 2 Tbsp. curry paste

- 4 Tbsp. fish sauce

- 1 cup chopped onions

- 1 cup coconut milk

- 1 lime - juice & 1 cup chicken broth

- 1 cup chopped cilantro & 3 cloves garlic.

Directions::

1. Blend lime, onions, curry paste, cilantro and spices.
2. Put chicken and other Ingredients: in the slow cooker and pour blended Ingredients: over.

3. Cover, and cook on low for 8 hours.

4. Decorate with fresh basil leaves.

Chicken & Artichoke Hearts

Ingredients:

- 4 pounds chicken meat

- 2 cups chopped carrots.

- 8 Artichokes, tops sliced, trimmed

- 1 Tbsp. ground cumin.

- 1 cup chicken broth

- 2 cups chopped onions

- 2 tbsp. coconut oil

- Salt, ground black pepper to taste

Directions::

1. Put Ingredients: in the slow cooker.
2. Cover, and cook on low for 8 hours.

Green Peppers, Chicken And Green Onions

Ingredients:

- 4 pounds chopped chicken meat

- 2 cups sliced green peppers

- 2 Tbsp. minced garlic.

- 1 Tbsp. ground cumin.

- 2 cups chopped green onions

- 2 tbsp. coconut oil

- Salt, ground black pepper to taste

Directions::

1. Put Ingredients: in the slow cooker.
2. Cover, and cook on low for 8 hours.

Haitian Spinach Shrimp Stew

Ingredients:

- 1 tsp. dried red pepper flakes (to taste).

- 4 whole cloves (discard after cooking)

- 2 cups fish broth

- 1 cup tomato paste.

- 1 lime – juice only & 1/8 ground cloves

- 2 cups chopped onions

- 2 tbsp. coconut oil

- Salt, ground black pepper to taste

- 4 pounds shrimp

- 3 cups spinach leaves

Directions::

1. Put Ingredients: in the slow cooker.

2. Cover, and cook on low for 8 hours.

Black Bean Chicken Chili

Ingredients:

- 2 cups black beans

- 4 fresh hot chili peppers, chopped

- 2 tbsp. coconut oil

- 2 onions, chopped

- 3 cloves garlic, minced

- 2 pounds cubed chicken meat

- 2 cups diced red and yellow peppers

- 2 cups sliced celery

- 1 cup tomato paste

- 2 cups chicken broth

- 1 tbsp. cumin seeds

- 1 tsp. dried oregano

- 1 tsp. ground cayenne pepper

- 1 tsp. ground coriander

- 1 tsp. salt

Directions::

1. Put Ingredients: in the slow cooker.

2. Cover, and cook on low for 8 hours.

Duck Curry

Ingredients:

- Curry Paste, but go low on the heat

- 1 tsp. paprika

- 1/2 cup coconut milk or cream

- Cilantro for garnishing

- 1 small chopped onion

- 1 chopped carrot

- 1 zucchini, sliced in 2 inch slices

- 2 tbsp. coconut oil

- 4 pounds duck meat

Directions::

1. Make Curry Paste. Add the chicken, veggies and the cream.
2. Stir to combine, add to crockpot & cook on low for 8 hours.

Tandoori Paneer Tikka Masala

Ingredients:

- 1 (2 inch) piece fresh ginger root, chopped

- 5 cloves garlic, chopped

For The Kebabs:

- 1 teaspoon cayenne pepper, or to taste

- 16 ounces paneer, cut into 1-inch cubes

- 1 green bell pepper, cut in 1-inch pieces

- 1 red bell pepper, cut in 1-inch pieces

- 1 large onion, cut into 1-inch pieces

- 1 cup plain yogurt

- 2 tablespoons mustard oil

- 1 lime, juiced

- 2 teaspoons dried fenugreek leaves

- 1 teaspoon garam masala

For The Sauce:

- 2 large tomatoes, finely chopped

- 1 lime, juiced

- 1 tablespoon ground coriander

- 1 teaspoon cayenne pepper, or to taste

- 1 teaspoon ground turmeric

- salt to taste

- 1 cup cashews

- 2 tablespoons olive oil

- 2 teaspoons cumin seeds

- 1 onion, finely chopped

- 1 tablespoon dried fenugreek leaves

- 1 teaspoon garam masala

Directions:

1. Soak 8 to 10 wooden skewers in water while you prepare the kebabs.

2. Process garlic and ginger in a food processor until a smooth paste forms.

3. Combine yogurt, mustard oil, lime juice of 1/2 lime, 1 1/2 teaspoons fenugreek leaves, 1 teaspoon garam masala, 1/2 teaspoon cayenne, and 1/2 of the ginger-garlic paste in a bowl. Whisk until smooth.

4. Add paneer, green bell pepper, red bell pepper, and onion. Stir until coated.

5. Preheat the oven to 400 degrees F (200 degrees C).

6. Thread the coated paneer, peppers, and onion onto the soaked skewers.

7. Place kebabs in a baking dish.

8. Bake in the preheated oven until kebabs are golden brown, 25 to 30 minutes.

9. Soak cashews in a bowl of hot water for 10 minutes; blend as finely or coarsely as desired.

10. Heat olive oil in a large saucepan over medium-high heat.

11. Add cumin seeds; cook until sputtering, about 1 minute.

12. Add remaining onion; cook and stir until translucent, about 5 minutes.

13. Add the remaining ginger-garlic paste, 1 tablespoon fenugreek leaves, and 1/2 teaspoon garam masala.

14. Cook and stir until flavors blend, about 2 minutes.

15. Stir in tomatoes; cover and cook until tomatoes break down, about 5 minutes.

16. Stir the ground cashews into the saucepan with the tomato mixture.

17. Add juice of 1/2 lime, coriander, 1 teaspoon cayenne, turmeric, and salt.

18. Let simmer until sauce is thickened, adding some water if sauce gets too dry and sticks to the pan, about 5 minutes more.

19. Add the baked kebabs to the sauce. Stir to coat evenly.

20. If you don't like to make a sauce, you can serve the tikka by itself on a bed of onions and lime wedges.

21. You can use 2 tablespoons of store-bought ginger-garlic paste instead of making your own.

Tandoori Masala Spice Mix

Ingredients:

- 1 teaspoon ground mace

- 1 teaspoon ground fenugreek

- 1 teaspoon ground cinnamon

- 1 teaspoon ground black pepper

- 1 teaspoon ground cardamom

- 1 teaspoon ground nutmeg

- 2 tablespoons ground coriander

- 2 tablespoons ground cumin

- 1 teaspoon garlic powder

- 1 teaspoon ground ginger

- 1 teaspoon ground cloves

Directions:

1. Combine coriander, cumin, garlic powder, ginger, cloves, mace, fenugreek, cinnamon, black pepper, cardamom, and nutmeg together in a bowl; store in an airtight container.

Tandoori Masala Spice Mix

Ingredients:

- 1 teaspoon ground fenugreek

- 1 teaspoon ground cinnamon

- 1 teaspoon ground black pepper

- 1 teaspoon ground cardamom

- 1 teaspoon ground nutmeg

- 2 tablespoons ground coriander

- 2 tablespoons ground cumin

- 1 teaspoon garlic powder

- 1 teaspoon ground ginger

- 1 teaspoon ground cloves

- 1 teaspoon ground mace

Directions:

1. Combine coriander, cumin, garlic powder, ginger, cloves, mace, fenugreek, cinnamon, black pepper, cardamom, and nutmeg together in a bowl; store in an airtight container.

Masala Beef With Ginger And Curry Leaf

Ingredients:

- 1 (1 1/2 inch) piece fresh ginger root, grated

- 6 cloves garlic, minced

- 1 teaspoon ground turmeric

- 1 teaspoon salt

- 1 cup coconut oil

- 1/2 teaspoon whole mustard seeds

- 4 fresh curry leaves

- 3 teaspoons lemon juice

- 1 teaspoon ground black pepper

- 3 bay leaves

- 1 (1 inch) piece cinnamon stick

- 5 cardamom pods

- 4 whole cloves

- 2 teaspoons fennel seeds

- 10 whole black peppercorns

- 2 pounds beef tenderloin, cubed

- 3 cups chopped onion, divided

- 5 green chile peppers, halved lengthwise

Directions:

1. To make the masala powder: Grind the bay leaves, cinnamon, cardamom, cloves, fennel seeds and peppercorns in a spice grinder until mixture is a fine powder.

2. Place the beef cubes, masala powder, 2 cups chopped onion, green chiles, grated fresh ginger, garlic and turmeric in a large, heavy pot.

3. Add water to cover (about 1 cup) and bring to a boil.

4. Reduce heat and simmer for 30 minutes until beef is cooked through. Add salt.

5. Stir and continue to simmer about 10 minutes or until mixture is almost dry, but do not allow it to burn (add a bit more water, if necessary). Set aside.

6. Heat oil in a large skillet over medium-high heat.

7. Add mustard seeds and cook until they begin to pop.

8. Immediately add remaining 1 cup chopped onion and stir over medium heat until onions soften and begin to brown, about 10 to 12 minutes.

9. Add curry leaves and cook until brown, about 3 minutes.

10. Stir in the beef mixture, black pepper, and lemon juice.

11. Cook until nicely browned and heated through, about 8 minutes.

12. You can adjust the spiciness of this recipe by increasing or decreasing the number of green chiles.

13. Also, you can remove the green chiles before serving, if desired.

Jonagold's Chicken Vindaloo

Ingredients:

- 8 dried curry leaves

- 1 teaspoon black mustard seeds

- 1/2 cup water

- 1 quart vegetable oil for frying

- 1 large potato, peeled and cut into 1 inch pieces

- 2 tablespoons distilled white vinegar

- 2 pounds skinless chicken drumsticks

- 5 tablespoons vegetable oil

- 2 onions, finely chopped

- 4 large cloves garlic, minced

- 1 inch piece fresh ginger root, minced

- 3 tablespoons distilled white vinegar

- 1 teaspoon ground coriander

- 1 teaspoon ground cumin

- 1 teaspoon garam masala

- 1 teaspoon ground black pepper

- salt to taste

- 1 teaspoon ground turmeric

- 1 teaspoon cayenne pepper

Directions:

1. Cut a few shallow slits into each chicken drumstick, and place into a resealable plastic bag; set aside.
2. Heat 5 tablespoons of vegetable oil in a Dutch oven or large pot over medium-high heat.
3. Stir in the onion, garlic, and ginger.
4. Cook and stir until the onion has turned golden brown, about 7 minutes.

5. Remove the pot from the heat, and use a slotted spoon to scoop the onion mixture into a blender.

6. Leave as much oil in the pot as you can, and set aside.

7. Add 3 tablespoons white vinegar, coriander, cumin, garam masala, black pepper, salt, turmeric, and cayenne pepper.

8. Puree until smooth, then pour into the bag with the chicken; mix until the chicken is evenly coated, and squeeze out excess air.

9. Marinate at room temperature for 1 hour, or in the refrigerator for 3 hours or longer.

10. After the chicken has marinated, heat the oil left in the Dutch oven over high heat, and stir in the curry leaves and mustard seeds.

11. Once the mustard seeds have finished popping and have turned gray, remove the chicken from its marinade, and cook until browned on all sides, about 5 minutes.

12. Pour in the remaining marinade and water.

13. Bring to a simmer, then reduce heat to medium-low, cover, and simmer 20 minutes.

14. Heat oil in a deep-fryer or large saucepan to 375 degrees F (190 degrees C).

15. While the chicken is cooking, deep fry the potato cubes until golden brown.

16. Drain on a paper towel-lined plate.

17. Once the chicken has cooked for 20 minutes, stir in the potatoes and 2 tablespoons of white vinegar.

18. Recover, and continue to simmer until the chicken is no longer pink at the bone, at least more 10 minutes.

19. We have determined the nutritional value of oil for deep frying based on a retention value of 10% after cooking.

20. The exact amount will vary depending on cooking time and temperature, ingredient density, and the specific type of oil used.

Grilled Chicken Thighs Tandoori

Ingredients:

- 4 teaspoons paprika

- 2 teaspoons ground cumin

- 2 teaspoons ground cinnamo

- 2 teaspoons ground coriander

- 16 chicken thighs

- olive oil spray

- 2 (6 ounce) containers plain yogurt

- 2 teaspoons kosher salt

- 1 teaspoon black pepper

- 1 teaspoon ground cloves

- 2 tablespoons freshly grated ginger

- 3 cloves garlic, minced

Directions:

1. In a medium bowl, stir together yogurt, salt, pepper, cloves, and ginger.

2. Mix in garlic, paprika, cumin, cinnamon, and coriander. Set aside.

3. Rinse chicken under cold water, and pat dry with paper towels.

4. Place chicken in a large resealable plastic bag.

5. Pour yogurt mixture over chicken, press air out of bag, and seal.

6. Turn the bag over several times to distribute marinade.

7. Place bag in a bowl, and refrigerate 8 hours, or overnight, turning bag occasionally.

8. Preheat an outdoor grill for direct medium heat.

9. Remove chicken from bag, and discard marinade.

10. With paper towels, wipe off excess marinade.

11. Spray chicken pieces with olive oil spray.

12. Place chicken on the grill, and cook about 2 minutes.

13. Turn, and cook 2 minutes more. Then arrange

14. the chicken to receive indirect heat, and cook approximately 35 to 40 minutes, to an internal temperature of 180 degrees F.

Indian Tandoori Chicken

Ingredients:

- 1 teaspoon cayenne pepper

- 1 teaspoon yellow food coloring

- 1 teaspoon red food coloring

- 2 teaspoons finely chopped cilantro

- 1 lemon, cut into wedges

- 2 pounds chicken, cut into pieces

- 1 teaspoon salt

- 1 lemon, juiced

- 2 cups plain yogurt

- 1 onion, finely chopped

- 1 clove garlic, minced

- 1 teaspoon grated fresh ginger root

- 2 teaspoons garam masala

Directions:

1. Remove skin from chicken pieces, and cut slits into them lengthwise.
2. Place in a shallow dish.
3. Sprinkle both sides of chicken with salt and lemon juice. Set aside 20 minutes.
4. In a medium bowl, combine yogurt, onion, garlic, ginger, garam masala, and cayenne pepper.
5. Mix until smooth. Stir in yellow and red food coloring.
6. Spread yogurt mixture over chicken.
7. Cover, and refrigerate for 6 to 24 hours (the longer the better).
8. Preheat an outdoor grill for medium high heat, and lightly oil grate.
9. Cook chicken on grill until no longer pink and juices run clear.
10. Garnish with cilantro and lemon wedges.

11. This dish can also be baked in a hot oven (450 degrees F) for 25 to 30 minutes, or until chicken is done.

Tandoori Paneer Tikka Masala

Ingredients:

For The Ginger-Garlic Paste:

- 1 (2 inch) piece fresh ginger root, chopped

- 5 cloves garlic, chopped

For The Kebabs:

- 16 ounces paneer, cut into 1-inch cubes

- 1 green bell pepper, cut in 1-inch pieces

- 1 red bell pepper, cut in 1-inch pieces

- 1 large onion, cut into 1-inch pieces

- 1 cup plain yogurt

- 2 tablespoons mustard oil

- 1 lime, juiced

- 2 teaspoons dried fenugreek leaves

- 1 teaspoon garam masala

- 1 teaspoon cayenne pepper, or to taste

For The Sauce:

- 2 large tomatoes, finely chopped

- 1 lime, juiced

- 1 tablespoon ground coriander

- 1 teaspoon cayenne pepper, or to taste

- 1 teaspoon ground turmeric

- salt to taste

- 1 cup cashews

- 2 tablespoons olive oil

- 2 teaspoons cumin seeds

- 1 onion, finely chopped

- 1 tablespoon dried fenugreek leaves

- 1 teaspoon garam masala

Directions:

1. Soak 8 to 10 wooden skewers in water while you prepare the kebabs.

2. Process garlic and ginger in a food processor until a smooth paste forms.

3. Combine yogurt, mustard oil, lime juice of 1/2 lime, 1 1/2 teaspoons fenugreek leaves, 1 teaspoon garam masala, 1/2 teaspoon cayenne, and 1/2 of the ginger-garlic paste in a bowl. Whisk until smooth.

4. Add paneer, green bell pepper, red bell pepper, and onion. Stir until coated.

5. Preheat the oven to 400 degrees F (200 degrees C).

6. Thread the coated paneer, peppers, and onion onto the soaked skewers.

7. Place kebabs in a baking dish.

8. Bake in the preheated oven until kebabs are golden brown, 25 to 30 minutes.

9. Soak cashews in a bowl of hot water for 10 minutes; blend as finely or coarsely as desired.

10. Heat olive oil in a large saucepan over medium-high heat.

11. Add cumin seeds; cook until sputtering, about 1 minute.

12. Add remaining onion; cook and stir until translucent, about 5 minutes.

13. Add the remaining ginger-garlic paste, 1 tablespoon fenugreek leaves, and 1/2 teaspoon garam masala.

14. Cook and stir until flavors blend, about 2 minutes.

15. Stir in tomatoes; cover and cook until tomatoes break down, about 5 minutes.

16. Stir the ground cashews into the saucepan with the tomato mixture.

17. Add juice of 1/2 lime, coriander, 1 teaspoon cayenne, turmeric, and salt.

18. Let simmer until sauce is thickened, adding some water if sauce gets too dry and sticks to the pan, about 5 minutes more.

19. Add the baked kebabs to the sauce. Stir to coat evenly.

20. If you don't like to make a sauce, you can serve the tikka by itself on a bed of onions and lime wedges.

21. You can use 2 tablespoons of store-bought ginger-garlic paste instead of making your own.

Root Vegetable, Barley, Kale & Sausage Stew (Paleo)

Ingredients:

- 2 cup. Vegetable Stock

- 4 Handfuls Of Kale

- 1 Tsp. Of Wholegrain Mustard

- Salt And Pepper

- Sprinkling Of Fresh Chives

- 1 Rutabaga, Chopped

- 2 Carrots, Chopped

- 1 Onion, Chopped

- 5 Pork And Sage Chipolata Sausages

- 2 Garlic Cloves

Directions:

1. Add the vegetables and half the stock to pot and simmer for half an hour as you brown the sausage.
2. Crumble the sausage in food processor and add to the slow cooker.
3. Add the vegetable stock and vegetables to the food processor and pulse until it's a puree.
4. Add that to the slow cooker along with the remainder of the Ingredients:.
5. Cook on low for six hours.

Crockpot Jambalaya Soup (Paleo)

Ingredients:

- Cajun Seasoning

- 3 Tbsp. Paprika

- 2 Tbsp. Salt

- 2 Tbsp. Garlic Powder

- 1 Tbsp. Pepper

- 1 Tbsp. Onion Powder

- 1 Tbsp. Cayenne Pepper

- 1 Tbsp. Dried Oregano

- 1 Tbsp. Dried Thyme

- 5 cup. Chicken Stock.

- 4 Peppers, Chopped

- 1 Onion, Chopped

- 15 oz. Diced Tomatoes

- 2 Garlic Cloves, Diced

- 2 Bay Leafs

- 1 Lb. Large Shrimp

- 4 Oz. Chicken, Diced

- 1 Package Spicy Andouille Sausage

- 1 Head Of Cauliflower

- 2 cup. Okra

- 3 Tbsp. Cajun Seasoning

- 1/2 cup. Frank's Red Hot

Directions:

1. Put the peppers through the bay leafs in the slow cooker with the stock.
2. Set the slow cooker too low for six hours.
3. Half an hour before it's finished, put in the sausages.

4. While it cooks, make some cauliflower rice by pulsing it in a food processor until it resembles rice.
5. During the last twenty minutes, add the rice and raw shrimp.

Perfectly Cooked Yams (Paleo)

Ingredients:

- 5 Medium Sweet Potatoes Or Yams

Directions:

1. Wrap the potatoes or yams in foil and put them in slow cooker on low for eight hours or four hours on high.

Pulled Pork Waffle Burgers (Paleo)

Ingredients:

- 3 Eggs, Whisked

- 1 cup. Canned Coconut Milk

- 2 Tbsp. Bacon Fat

- 3 Pieces Of Bacon, Cooked And Chopped

- 2 Tbsp. Chives, Finely Chopped

- 5-6 Pieces Of Bacon, Cooked

- Slice Pickles

- 2 Lbs. Pork Butt

- 1 Tbsp. Garlic Powder

- 1 Yellow Onion, Sliced

- Salt And Pepper

- 1 Tsp. Onion Powder

- 2 cup. Avocado Oil

- 1 Egg

- 1 Tsp. Lemon Juice

- 1 Tsp. Dijon Mustard

- 1/2 Tsp. Garlic Powder

- Salt And Pepper, To Taste

- 1 Tsp. Maple Syrup

- 2 cup. Almond Flour

- 1 Tsp. Baking Soda

- 1 Tsp. Garlic Powder

- Salt And Pepper, To Taste

Directions:

1. Put the roast in a slow cooker. Add the onions, garlic and onion powder, and the salt and pepper.

2. Cover and cook six to eight hours on low or until it's very tender and falls apart.

3. Once the pork's done, shred it in the slow cooker.
4. Now make the mayonnaise so that you can chill it in the refrigerator.
5. Put the avocado oil through the salt and pepper in a tall container and put the immersion blender in the bottom of the container.
6. Turn it on and wait for the mixture to thicken.
7. When it's thick, pour in the maple syrup and fold that in with a spoon.
8. Put in the refrigerator to allow it to cool.
9. To make the waffles, mix the almond flour through the salt and pepper.
10. Add the eggs through the chives and mix will to combine.
11. Heat up your waffle iron and pour the mix into the center of the waffle area. Cook until crispy.

12. When the waffles are done, put one on a plate, layer with mayonnaise, pork, bacon, pickles, mayonnaise, and another waffle.

Crockpot Sweet Potato Basil Soup (Paleo)

Ingredients:

- 2 Garlic Cloves, Minced

- 1 Tbsp. Dried Basil

- Salt And Pepper

- 2 Sweet Potatoes Or Yams, Diced

- 1 Yellow Onion, Sliced

- 1 (14oz) Can Of Coconut Milk

- 1 cup. Vegetable Broth

Directions:

1. Put all the Ingredients: in a slow cooker.
2. Mix it around thoroughly.
3. Cook for three hours on high.
4. Use a blender and puree the mix until it's smooth.

Sausage And Peppers

Ingredients:

- 1/2 tsp crushed red pepper flakes

- 1 28oz can crushed tomatoes

- 1/2 cup water

- 2 lbs uncooked Italian sausage links

- 2 yellow onions, thinly sliced

- 4 green peppers, thinly sliced

- 6 cloves garlic, minced

- 1 Tbsp salt

- 1 tsp Italian seasoning

- 1/2 tsp oregano

Directions:

1. Add onions, peppers, and garlic to the slow cooker.

2. Add salt, Italian seasoning, oregano, red pepper, tomatoes, and water.

3. Stir together to distribute the seasonings and place the sausages on top.

4. Cook on low for 6 hours and serve hot.

Sausage Breakfast Casserole

Ingredients:

- 8 eggs

- 1 sweet potato, shredded

- 2 cup beef sausage, browned

- 2 Tbsp coconut oil

- 1 cup of sliced green onions/leeks

- 1 clove garlic, minced

- 1 cup kale, chopped

Directions:

1. Heat coconut oil in a skillet over medium-high heat.
2. When the oil is hot, add the green onions, garlic, and kale and sauté for 3 - 4 minutes. Add to a large bowl.
3. Add the eggs, sweet potato, and beef sausage to the vegetables in the bowl. Stir together.

4. Pour the bowl into the slow cooker and cook on low for 6 hours.
5. Sprinkle salt and pepper to taste on top and allow to cool and become stable before serving.

Sausage Ratatouille

Ingredients:

- 1 onion, sliced

- 4 cloves garlic, minced

- 1 25oz jar pasta sauce (either find one that doesn't have a lot of additives or else make your own)

- 1 tsp salt

- 2 tsp dried basil

- 1 lb Italian sausage (not in casing), uncooked

- 1 red bell pepper, diced

- 1 large eggplant, cubed

- 1 lbs zucchini, cubed

Directions:

1. Prepare your vegetables and add to the slow cooker.

121

2. Add the sausage making sure that the sausage is in evenly sized pieces.

3. Add pasta sauce, salt, and dried basil.

4. Cook on high for 4 hours.

5. Serve and enjoy, this dish is a meal in itself!

Rosemary And Thyme Roast Lamb

Ingredients:

- 4 sprigs thyme, stripped from the stalk

- 4 sprigs fresh rosemary, chopped

- 2 carrots, peeled and chopped

- 2 potatoes, peeled and chopped

- 3-4 lbs boneless lamb roast

- 2 Tbsp olive oil

- Salt and pepper

- 1 cup chicken broth

- 4 cloves garlic, minced

Directions:

1. Heat a cast iron skillet to medium-high heat with the olive oil.

2. Sprinkle salt and pepper generously over the lamb roast and then sear each side of the roast, which will take 3-4 minutes per side.

3. Transfer the roast to the slow cooker and then pour the chicken broth into the skillet and stir, being sure to scrape up the browned bits from the bottom of the pan.

4. Pour on top of the lamb in the slow cooker.

5. Add the garlic, thyme, and rosemary to the roast and cook for 8 hours on low.

6. Half way through the cooking, add the carrots and potatoes.

7. When the 8 hour mark is hit, make sure it is tender to your liking and enjoy!

Moroccan Lamb Stew

Ingredients:

- 1 tsp ginger

- 1 tsp coriander

- 1 tsp cayenne pepper

- 1 cup vegetable or chicken stock

- 1 14oz can diced tomatoes (drained)

- 1 cup chopped dried prunes or dried apricots

- 1/4 cup slivered almonds (optional)

- 3 lbs lamb, cut into 1 inch cubes

- 2 onions, chopped

- 4 Tbsp coconut oil

- 4 cloves garlic, minced

- 2 tsp cumin

- 1 tsp cinnamon

Directions:

1. (Optional, you can just add the meat to the slow cooker directly) Heat 2 Tbsp of coconut oil to medium-high heat in a skillet and then add the lamb pieces.

2. Sprinkle with salt and pepper and let cook for 2- 3 minutes to brown the sides.

3. Move to the slow cooker and then add the other 2 Tbsp coconut oil to sauté the onions and garlic. Add onion to the slow cooker.

4. Once the lamb, onions, and garlic are in the slow cooker, add the cumin, cinnamon, ginger, coriander, pepper, stock, tomatoes, and dried fruit.

5. Cook on low for 6 hours and serve warm with toasted almonds on top.

6. Goes great as a stew or on top of cauliflower rice or mashed sweet potatoes.

Indian Curried Lamb

Ingredients:

- 1 Tbsp tomato paste

- 1 Tbsp red curry powder

- 2 tsp garam masala powder

- 1 tsp tumeric powder

- 1 tsp fennel seeds

- 1 cup coconut milk

- 1 Tbsp coconut oil

- 2 lbs diced lamb

- 1 yellow onion

- 2 cloves garlic, diced

- 1 cup water

- 1 stalk celery, diced

- 1 carrot, diced

Directions:

1. In a cast iron pan or other skillet, heat coconut oil until medium-high heat.

2. Add the lamb and cook 2-3 minutes on each side until just brown.

3. Add the onion and garlic to the skillet and cook for an additional 2-3 minutes until they begin to start turning more translucent.

4. Turn off the heat on the skillet and add the lamb, onion, and garlic to the slow cooker.

5. Add water, diced celery and carrots, tomato paste, curry powder, masala powder, tumeric powder and fennel seeds. Cook on low for 6 hours.

6. In the last hour of cooking, add the coconut milk and stir to combine.

7. Once all of the vegetables and lamb are tender, serve warm.

8. There will be plenty of sauce which will make a great accompaniment to your favorite vegetables.

Spiced Stuffed Apples

Ingredients:

- 2 Tbsp cinnamon

- 1 tsp nutmeg

- 1 tsp salt

- 1 cup water

- Diced nuts (optional)

- 4 large green apples

- 1 cup coconut butter

- 1/2 cup nut butter (almond butter, peanut butter, even sunbutter)

Directions:

1. Combine the coconut butter, nut butter, cinnamon, nutmeg, and salt.
2. Core the apples leaving the bottom intact if possible.
3.
4. If you have a corer, this is simpler but if not then use a knife and/or spoon to remove the core.
5. Pour the water into the slow cooker and place the cored apples into the slow cooker.
6. Distribute the butter mix between the apples until each is filled.
7. Top the apples with additional cinnamon and cook for 2 - 3 hours.
8. Cooking for less time will give you a crunchier experience so adjust to your liking.
9. If desired, top with diced nuts to give the dessert some additional texture.

Pumpkin Pudding

Ingredients:

- 3 eggs

- 1 cup natural sweetener (honey or maple syrup - you can use less if you don't like things too sweet or aren't going to be working off the calories)

- 2 tsp pumpkin pie spice

- 2 Tbsp vanilla extract

- 3 Tbsp coconut flour

- 1 tsp baking powder

- 3 Tbsp coconut oil

- 2 cups pureed pumpkin

- 2 cups coconut milk

Directions:

1. Use a paper towel to apply the coconut oil around the sides and bottom of the slow cooker to prevent sticking.

2. In a separate bowl, combine the pumpkin, coconut milk, eggs, sweetener, pumpkin pie spice, vanilla, coconut flour, and baking powder.

3. Use beaters, a blender, or just lots of muscle to get it smooth.

4. Pour into the slow cooker and cook for 8 hours.

5. A crust will form on top but the base will have a pudding consistency.

6. If you want to add some texture, add nuts or dried fruit on top.

Berry Crumble

Ingredients:

- 1 cup almond flour

- 1 Tbsp honey

- 3 cups fresh or frozen mixed berries (we like raspberries, strawberries, blackberries and blueberries)

- 4 Tbsp coconut oil

Directions:

1. Spread the berries around the base of the slow cooker and top with 1 Tbsp of coconut oil.
2. In a separate bowl, melt 2 Tbsp of coconut oil (will take just a couple seconds in a microwave) and then add the honey.
3. Stir in the almond flour and mix with a fork until it begins to clump.

4. Sprinkle the crumble over the berries in the slow cooker. Cook on low for 2 hours.
5. Serve warm, optionally with coconut milk ice cream.

Tomatoes And Kidney Beans

Ingredients:

- 7 Ounces of Sun Dried and Oil packed Tomatoes – Chopped and Drained

- 2 Ounces of Shaved Asiago Cheese

- 1/3 Cup of Pine Nuts

- 3 Cans of White Kidney Beans

- 1 Can of Vegetable Broth

- 3 Minced Garlic Cloves

Directions:

1. In a 4-quart cooker combine vegetables, beans, broth, and garlic.

2. Cover the mixture and cook it on low for 6-8 hours or on high for 4 hours.

3. Stir in tomatoes, if you have it on the low setting turn it to high when you add the tomatoes.

4. Cover it and cook it for 15 more minutes.

5. Serve it with the cheese sprinkled on top.

Chicken Tacos

Ingredients:

- Whole Wheat Flour Tortillas

- Shredded Cheddar Cheese

- Tomatoes – Diced

- Shredded Lettuce

- Sour Cream

- Salsa

- 2 Pounds of Boneless Chicken Breast

- 1 Can of Red Enchilada Sauce

- 1 Can of Diced Green Chilies

- 2 Cup of Diced red Onion

Directions:

1. Put the chicken, green chilies, enchilada sauce, and onion in the 4-quart cooker.

2. Cook on high for 3 – 5 hrs.

3. Shred the chicken with forks.

4. Serve on the tortilla and add lettuce, sour cream, cheese, and tomatoes.

Chicken Creole

Ingredients:

- 3 Minced Cloves of Garlic

- 1 Diced white Onion

- 1 – 4 Ounce of Drained button Mushrooms

- 1 Jalapeno Pepper – Chopped

- 4 Boneless Chicken Breasts

- Dash of Salt and Pepper

- Creole Seasoning

- 1 – 14.5 Ounces of Stewed Tomatoes

- 1 Diced Celery Stalk

- 1 Diced Green Bell Pepper

Directions:

1. Put the chicken breasts in the cooker.

2. Season with pepper, salt, and the Creole seasoning.
3. Stir in the tomatoes with the liquid, bell pepper, celery, garlic, onion, jalapeno pepper, and mushrooms.
4. Cook it on low for 10-12 hours or 5-6 hours on high.

Mu Shu Turkey

Ingredients:

- 1/2 tsp. of Cinnamon

- 1 Pound of Boneless Turkey Breast – Cut into strips.

- 6 – 7 inch Flour Tortillas

- 3 Cups of Coleslaw Mix

- 1 Can of Drained and Pitted Plums

- 1 Cup of Orange Juice

- 1/2 Cup of Chopped red Onion

- 1 Tbsp. of Fresh Ginger

Directions:

1. Put the plums in a food processor and blend them until they are smooth.

2. Combine the orange juice, plums, onion, cinnamon, and ginger into a 4-quart cooker.

3. Put the turkey on the plum mixture and cook it for 3-4 hours.
4. Remove the turkey and put it in the tortillas.
5. Spoon 2 tablespoons of the plum sauce on the turkey.
6. Top it with 1 cup of coleslaw mix.

Chicken Casserole

Ingredients:

- 1 Can of Beef Broth – Fat Free

- 1 Can of Cream of Mushroom Soup – 98% Fat Free

- 4 Ounces of Drained Mushrooms

- 2 Pounds of Boneless Chicken Breasts – Cubed

- 1 Package of Onion Soup Mix

Directions:

1. Put all Ingredients: into a 3-quart slow cooker.
2. Cover and cook the chicken for 8-10 hours on low or 3-4 hours on high.
3. Serve it on rice or noodles.

Minestrone Stew

Ingredients:

- 2 Bay Leaves

- 4 Cups of Vegetable Stock

- 2 Cups of Water

- 3 Cups of Tomato Juice

- 1 Can of Red Kidney Beans – Drained, Rinsed

- 1 Can of Cannellii Beans – Drained, Rinsed

- 2 Cups of Zucchini – Diced

- 1 Cup of Tubular Pasta

- 1 Can of Green Beans – Drained

- 1 Can of Tomatoes – Diced

- 2 Cups of Carrots – Chopped

- 2 Cups of Potatoes – Chopped

- 2 Cups of Celery – Chopped

- 1 White Onion – Diced

- 3-4 Cloves of Garlic – Minced

- 1 Tbsp. of Italian Seasoning

- 1 tsp. of Salt

- 1 tsp. of Pepper

Directions:

1. Place the carrots, tomatoes, potatoes, onion, celery, garlic, salt, pepper, bay leaves, and Italian seasoning in the cooker.
2. Add in the stock, V8, and water.
3. Cook it for 6-8 hours on low or 3-4 hours on high.
4. After it cooks, add in the kidney beans, the cannellii beans, green beans, zucchini, and the pasta.
5. Cook it on high for another 15 minutes.

Green Chili Stuffed Chicken Breasts

Ingredients:

- 1 teaspoon chili powder

- salt and pepper to taste

- 1 can cream of mushroom soup

- 1 cup hot enchilada sauce

- 4 boneless, skinned chicken breast halves, pounded thin

- 3 ounces cream cheese

- 3/4 cups shredded Cheddar or Monterey Jack cheese

- 4 ounces green chilies

Directions:

1. Mix cream cheese, shredded cheese, chiles, chili powder and salt and pepper in a bowl.

2. Flatten chicken breasts and divide the mixture into 4 parts and place on each chicken breast.

3. Roll up the chicken breasts.

4. Lay the chicken rolls in the slow cooker, with seam-side down.

5. Top chicken breast rolls with remaining cheese mixture, soup, and enchilada sauce.

6. Cover and cook on LOW for 6 to 7 hours.

Honeyed Chicken Wings

Ingredients:

- 2 tbsp. vegetable oil

- 2 tbsp. ketchup

- 1 garlic clove, minced

- 3 lb. chicken wings

- Salt & pepper, to taste

- 1 c. honey

- 1 c. soy sauce

Directions:

1. Discard chicken wing tips.
2. Cut each wing into 2 pieces and season with salt and pepper.
3. Mix remaining Ingredients: and mix well.
4. Lay wings in slow cooker and pour sauce over.
5. Cook 6 to 8 hours on low.

Lemon Tarragon Chicken

Ingredients:

- 1 package frozen asparagus

- 2 tablespoons flour

- 1 cup heavy or whipping cream

- salt and pepper to taste

- 1 pound frozen chicken breasts, boneless

- 1/2 cup lemon juice

- 1/2 cup chicken stock

- 1 teaspoon tarragon (dried)

Directions:

1. Place frozen chicken breasts in Crock Pot and add lemon juice, broth, and tarragon.
2. Cook on low 6 hours. Add in asparagus.
3. Mix cream and flour together and add.
4. Cook another hour on high.

5. Serve over noodles or rice.

Low-Fat Chicken & Veggie Bake

Ingredients:

- 1 bottle fat free Italian salad dressing

- 1 packaged frozen veggies

- 1 can water chestnuts (optional)

- salt & pepper

- 8 boneless, skinless chicken breasts

- 2 cans whole potatoes, drained

- 1 tsp garlic powder

Directions:

1. Season chicken breasts with salt, pepper and garlic.

2. Place chicken in bottom of slow cooker/Crock Pot.

3. Add remaining Ingredients:.

150

4. Cook on high for 4-6 hours or on low for 8-10 hours.

Maple Barbecue Chicken

Ingredients:

- 2 tsp. lemon juice

- 1 tsp. chili powder

- 1/2 tsp. garlic powder

- 4 boneless, skinned chicken breasts

- 1 c. ketchup

- 1 c. maple flavored syrup

- 2 tbsp. prepared mustard

- 2 tbsp. Worcestershire sauce

Directions:

1. Put all Ingredients: in slow cooker and cook on low for about 7 to 8 hours.

2. Take out the meat, shred and return to sauce.

3. Serve over hot rice.

Mediterranean Chicken

Ingredients:

- 1 tablespoon lemon juice

- 1 teaspoon oregano

- 1 onion, chopped

- 1 cup wine or brandy (optional)

- cooked rice

- Salt to taste

- 6 skinless and boneless chicken breasts

- 1 large can tomato sauce

- 1 small can tomato puree

- 1 can sliced mushrooms

- 1 can ripe olives, sliced or whole

- 1 tablespoon garlic

Directions:

1. Rinse and remove excess fat from chicken.

2. Mix all Ingredients: in the slow cooker, except the rice.

3. Cover and cook on low for 6 to 8 hours.

4. Serve chicken and sauce over rice.

One Pot Chicken Gravy

Ingredients:

- 1 packaged baby carrots

- 1 can cream of chicken soup

- 1 packaged dry onion soup mix

- Boneless, skinless chicken breasts

- Potatoes, quartered, with jackets

- About 6 stalks celery

Directions:

1. Lay the vegetables at the bottom of Crock Pot.
2. Brown chicken breasts in PAM or vegetable spray.
3. Lay the chicken over vegetables.
4. Pour the cream of chicken soup all over the chicken.
5. Sprinkle with dry onion soup mix.

6. Cover and cook 12 hours on low, or 6 hours on high.

Orange Burgundy Chicken

Ingredients:

- 1 cup dry red wine

- 2 tablespoons cornstarch

- 2 tablespoons brown sugar, packed

- 1 tablespoon lemon juice

- 1 teaspoon salt

- 3 to 3 pounds frying chicken, skinless and chopped up

- 1 cup orange marmalade

- 1 cup orange juice

Directions:

1. Wash the Chicken and place in slow cooker.
2. Mix remaining Ingredients: in a bowl and pour over chicken.
3. Cover and cook on low 6 to 8 hours.

4. Serve with rice and spinach salad.

Provincial Chicken

Ingredients:

- 2 teaspoons dried parsley flakes

- 1 teaspoon dried basil

- 1 tablespoon dried minced onion

- 1 cup shredded cheddar cheese

- 2 to 3 tablespoons sour cream (optional)

- hot noodles, rice or pasta

- 2 pounds chicken tenders, frozen

- 2 small zucchini, diced

- 1 can (4 oz) sliced black olives

- 1 tablespoon sherry wine vinegar or balsamic vinegar

- 1 can good-quality diced tomatoes (about 15 ounces)

- 1 can (10 oz) cream of chicken soup with herbs

Directions:

1. Mix first 9 Ingredients: in a slow cooker.

2. Cover and cook on low for 6 to 8 hours.

3. Put in the cheese and sour cream during the last 15 minutes.

4. Serve over hot noodles, rice or pasta.

Russian Chicken

Ingredients:

- 1 jar apricot preserves (10 oz.)

- 4 pieces chicken

- Seasoned salt and pepper to taste

- 1 bottle Russian dressing (16 oz.)

- 1 envelope onion soup mix

Directions:

1. MIx dressing, preserves and onion soup mix in bowl and pour into a slow cooker.
2. Season chicken with seasoned salt and pepper.
3. Lay the chicken, skin side down, in slow cooker.
4. Cook on LOW for 8 hours, or on HIGH for 4 hours.

Spaghetti Sauce With Chicken & Sausage

Ingredients:

- 1-2 tsp. Italian seasoning

- 2 (4 oz. each) cans mushroom stems and pieces, drained

- 2 jars favorite spaghetti sauce

- Hot cooked pasta

- 1 lb. Italian sausage

- 3-4 boneless chicken breasts, cut into 1-inch chunks

- 1 cup chopped green pepper

- 1 cup chopped onion

Directions:

1. In skillet, brown Italian sausage and take out.
2. Cut the Sausages into 1 to 2-inch chunks.
3. In same skillet, brown chicken pieces.

4. Lay the sausage and chicken in slow cooker.

5. Season with pepper, onion and Italian seasoning

6. Add mushrooms. Coat everything with Sauce.

7. Cover and cook on low for 6 to 8 hours.

8. Serve over spaghetti or other pasta.

Spanish Chicken

Ingredients:

- Sliced mushrooms, drained

- Stewed tomatoes

- Liquid to cover (beer, tomato soup or tomato sauce)

- 2 lb. boneless skinless chicken breast

- Seasoned salt & pepper to taste

- Black olives, pitted

Directions:

1. Chop chicken into bite-sized pieces and season it.
2. Put with remaining Ingredients: in slow cooker.
3. Cook all day on low. Serve over rice.

Spicy Chicken Wings

Ingredients:

- 1 c. melted butter

- 1 pkg. Hidden Valley Ranch original dry salad dressing mix

- 3 tbsp. vinegar

- 24 chicken wing drummettes

- 1/2 c. hot pepper sauce, or less

Directions:

1. Mix all Ingredients: together except chicken wings and salad dressing mix.
2. Place chicken wings in Crockpot.
3. Pour mixture over wings.
4. Sprinkle with dry dressing mix.
5. Sprinkle with paprika if you like.
6. Cook on low for 5 hours. Serve.

Sweet 'N' Sour Chicken

Ingredients:

- 3 split chicken breasts (remove skin, optional)

- 1 tsp. salt

- 1 (10 oz.) jar Sweet N Sour sauce

- 1 (15 oz.) can pineapple chunks, drained

- 2 tbsp. cornstarch

- 6 med. carrots, cut into 1/2" chunks

- 1 c. finely chopped green pepper

- 1 sm. onion, finely chopped

Directions:

1. Put all Ingredients: in slow cooker with chicken on top.
2. Cover and cook on low 6-8 hours.

3. Take out the chicken and thicken with 2 tablespoons cornstarch dissolved to a medium thick paste with water.
4. Pour over chicken breasts. Serve with rice.

Teriyaki Sauce Wings

Ingredients:

- 2 teaspoons ground ginger

- 2 cloves garlic, crushed

- 1/2 cup dry sherry

- 3 pounds chicken wings

- 1 onion, chopped

- 1 cup soy sauce

- 1 cup brown sugar

Directions:

1. Wash chicken, and pat dry. Discard wing tips.
2. Cut each wing at the joint.
3. Brown the wings on each side in a skillet.
4. Once browned, lay the chicken wings in a Crock Pot.
5. Combine all remaining Ingredients: together and pour over chicken wings.

6. Cook, covered, on low for 5 to 6 hours or on high for 2 to 3 hours.
7. Stir once or twice to keep wings coated with sauce. Serve.

Masala Beef & Rice

Ingredients:

- 2 cups water

- 3 garlic cloves, minced

- 16 ounces mixed vegetables

- 1 teaspoon each; ground turmeric, ginger, cinnamon, and black pepper

- 1 teaspoon each; seasoned salt and sea salt

- 1 tablespoon beef bouillon granules

- 2 tablespoons garam masala

- 3 pounds beef pot roast

- 2 cups cooked rice, warm

- 1 cup pine nuts, toasted

Directions:

1. In the slow cooker, add all Ingredients: except pine nuts and rice

2. Cover and cook for 8 hours on LOW setting

3. Sprinkle with pine nuts and enjoy with rice

Mediterranean Beef & Pasta

Ingredients:

- 1 tablespoon capers, drained

- 1 tablespoon balsamic vinegar

- 2 cups penne pasta

- 1 cup parmesan cheese, shredded

- 15 ounces diced tomatoes

- 14 ounces can artichoke hearts, drained, chopped

- 5 ounces jar mushrooms, drained, sliced

- 1 cup onion, chopped

- 1 pound beef stew meat

- 1 teaspoon sugar

- 1 teaspoon salt

- 1 teaspoon Italian seasoning

- 1 tablespoon garlic, dried, minced

Directions:

1. In the slow cooker, add beef, mushrooms, artichoke hearts, tomatoes, vinegar, capers, garlic, Italian seasoning, salt, onion, and sugar

2. Cover and cook for 7 hours on LOW

3. Following package direction, cook pasta until tender, drain and place in a bowl, add oil and pepper

4. Serve beef sauce with pasta and top with cheese

Beef, Zucchini, & Eggplant Stew

Ingredients:

- 1 teaspoon black pepper

- 1 teaspoon sage, dried

- 1 teaspoon thyme, dried

- 3 cups water

- 2 tablespoons mint, fresh, chopped

- 2 pounds lean beef, cut into cubes

- 1 pound chopped tomatoes

- 1 pound eggplant, cut into cubes

- 1 pound zucchini, sliced

- 2 onions, chopped

- 1 teaspoon salt

Directions:

1. In the slow cooker, add beef, eggplant, zucchini, onion, oil, tomatoes, sage, thyme, mint, salt, pepper, and water

2. Cover and cook for 6 hours on LOW

Herbed Beef Stew

Ingredients:

- 1 tablespoon grapeseed oil

- 1 teaspoon basil, dried

- 1 teaspoon parsley, dried

- 1 teaspoon oregano, dried

- 1 teaspoon cumin, ground

- 920 g beef, diced

- 75g Kalamata, pitted, chopped

- 420 g tin tomatoes, chopped

- 420 g tomato passata

- 420 g artichokes, drained

- 1 liter beef stock

- 4 garlic cloves, chopped

- 1 bay leaf

Directions:

1. Add oil in the skillet and heat over medium-high
2. Add beef and cook until evenly browned. Place into the slow cooker
3. Add all remaining Ingredients:
4. Cover and cook for 7 hours on LOW

Tuscan Beef Stew

Ingredients:

- 11 ounces can tomato soup

- 1 cup red wine

- 3 large carrots, peeled, diced

- 1 teaspoon garlic powder

- 1 teaspoon Italian seasoning, dried, crushed

- 2 pounds beef stew, cut into cubes

- 2 (15 ounces each) cans white cannellini beans, rinsed, drained

- 15 ounces diced tomatoes with basil, garlic and oregano

- 11ounces can beef broth

Directions:

1. In the slow cooker, add all Ingredients:
2. Cover and cook for 9 hours on LOW

Mediterranean Eggplant

Ingredients:

- 4 plum tomatoes, diced

- 1 tablespoon olive oil

- 2 teaspoons basil, dried

- 4 garlic cloves, peeled, minced

- 4 ounces feta cheese, crumbled

- 1 pound eggplant, peeled, diced

- 1 large red bell pepper, seeds removed, chopped

- 1 large zucchini, chopped

- 1 large onion, peeled, diced

Directions:

1. In the slow cooker, mix together all Ingredients: except feta

178

2. Cover and cook for 5 hours on LOW

3. Add cheese and serve

Greek Style Eggplant

Ingredients:

- 1 tablespoon extra-virgin olive oil

- 1 teaspoon black pepper

- 1 teaspoon turmeric, ground

- 1 teaspoon dry oregano

- 2 teaspoon coriander, ground

- 2 teaspoons sweet paprika

- Kosher salt, to taste

- 1 cup water

- 2 pounds eggplant, cut into cubes

- 1 green bell pepper, stemmed, diced

- 1 carrot, diced

- 2 bay leaves

180

- 6 garlic cloves, minced

- 1 yellow onion, diced

- 2 (15 ounces each) cans chickpeas

- 28 ounces can tomato, chopped

Directions:

1. In a large skillet, add oil and heat over medium-high
2. Add onions, carrots, and green pepper.
3. Cook for 3 minutes, stirring occasionally.
4. Stir in garlic, salt, bay leaf, paprika, coriander, oregano, turmeric, black pepper, and cinnamon.
5. Cook for 1 minute and transfer to the slow cooker
6. Add all remaining Ingredients:
7. Cover and cook for 4 hours on LOW

Lebanese Eggplant Stew

Ingredients:

- 1/2 cup parsley, fresh, chopped

- 1/2 cup olive oil

- 1 inch piece cinnamon

- 1 teaspoon allspice berries

- 1 teaspoon black peppercorns

- Salt, to taste

- 1/2 teaspoon red pepper flakes

- 1 large eggplant, peeled, cut into cubes

- 1 green bell pepper, stemmed, diced

- 3 tomatoes, quartered

- 3 garlic cloves, minced

- 1 onion, chopped

Directions:

1. In a food processor, add peppercorns, red pepper flakes, allspice berries, and cinnamon. Process until smooth. Keep aside

2. In the slow cooker, add all remaining Ingredients:.

3. Sprinkle with spice mix and add 1/2 cup of water or vegetable broth

4. Cover and cook for 4 hours on LOW

Eggplant & Tomato Sauce

Ingredients:

- 16 ounces can tomato paste

- 1 pound pasta

- 1 cup red wine

- 1 teaspoon oregano, dried

- Salt, to taste

- 1 medium eggplant, cut into cubes

- 2 garlic cloves, minced

- 1 onion, chopped

- 28 ounces can diced tomatoes, drained

Directions:

1. In the slow cooker, add all Ingredients: except pasta

2. Cover and cook for 6 hours on LOW

184

3. Cook pasta according to package direction and drain

4. Serve eggplant and tomato sauce with pasta

Italian Style Mushrooms

Ingredients:

- 1 teaspoon Italian seasoning

- 1 teaspoon sweet paprika

- 1 yellow onion, chopped

- 1 pounds mushrooms, halved

- 2 tablespoons olive oil

Directions:

1. In your Slow cooker, mix mushrooms with onion, olive oil, Italian seasoning, and paprika, toss, cover, and cook on Low for 4 hours.

2. Divide between plates and serve as a side dish.